Yoga for Parents

Mindfulness and Movement in Family Life

Table of Contents

Chapter 1. Introduction

Introducing our Special Report: "Yoga for Parents: Mindfulness and Movement in Family Life"! This beautifully composed guide will bring a dash of calmness and harmony to your bustling household. It isn't just another yoga manual; it's a distinctive blend of mindfulness and movement that both, parents and children, can resonate with. You'll learn how to incorporate yoga into your daily family life, turning ordinary moments into pathways for developing focus, strength, and balance. Loaded with fun and practical ideas, impressive visuals, and heartwarming testimonials, it will hook you from the turn of the first page. Embrace the chance to foster a healthier, happier family - all while enjoying some 'me-time'. Ready to embark on this illuminating journey? Let's unfurl those yoga mats and dive in!

Chapter 2. Setting the Stage: Introducing Yoga and Mindfulness to Your Family

Those initial moments leading to the introduction of yoga and mindfulness to your family can be both exciting and intimidating. However, rest assured that the steps recommended in this guide are designed to seamlessly integrate this lifestyle change into your day-to-day activities. These aren't meant to shock or disrupt, but rather to blend and harmonize. Above all, it's a process that maintains family unity and togetherness at its core. It's important to remember that yoga isn't just a series of poses - it's a philosophy, a way of life. And mindfulness is the icing on this holistic cake that can sweeten the quality of your family life.

2.1. The Importance of Yoga and Mindfulness in Family Life

Before we dive into the "how-tos", it's worth understanding why yoga and mindfulness matter for your family. Yoga and mindfulness go beyond physical benefits. The true beauty lies in their power to transform perspectives, relationships, and states of mind. Scientific studies have shown the ways these practices improve mental, emotional, and physical health. The tenets of patience, non-judgment, self-awareness, and gratitude that form their core can gift your family an environment that's healthy, nurturing, and joyful.

While yoga focuses on strength, flexibility, and balance in the physical realm, mindfulness brings the same qualities into our mental and emotional domains. A mindfulness approach enriches the yoga experience, as we become more aware and get in tune with our bodies. Together, yoga and mindfulness empower us to navigate life's ups and downs with greater equanimity.

2.2. Introducing Yoga

To bring yoga into your family's life, it's prudent to understand its essential components. Yoga is not merely about flexibility or striking impressive poses; rather, it's a philosophy of mind-body unity, breathing control, and self-awareness.

Yoga poses or 'asanas' enhance physical flexibility and strength. Coupled with 'pranayama' or breath control, these asanas enable us to govern our physiological responses better, naturally reducing stress. Don't be surprised to find a fun game of "Pose Pictionary" turning into an impromptu yoga session.

2.3. Introducing Mindfulness

Mindfulness is the practice of fully focusing on the present moment with openness and curiosity, without judgment. In the milieu of family life, it can translate to fully enjoying a meal together, having animated conversations during a hike, or even appreciating the tranquility during a quiet afternoon. For children, who naturally live in the moment, mindfulness can be an affirmation of their existing instincts.

2.4. Starting with Simple Poses and Noticing the Breath

As you start off, keep things light and fun. Begin with simple poses like 'Tree Pose' or 'Mountain Pose'. Focus not only on the posture but the breathing pattern involved. Teach your children to notice their breath – how it slows down or speeds up. The primary purpose is to cultivate awareness.

2.5. Cultivating a Mindful Attitude

Mindfulness is as simple as being completely present in the moment. Encourage open conversations about feelings and sensations during the yoga practice. This helps children identify and understand their emotions, helping them become emotionally savvy and fostering empathy.

2.6. Designing Your Yoga Space

Designating a family yoga space takes this commitment to the next level. An area that's clean, quiet, and comfortable, adorned with family pictures, plants, or favorite blankets allows your family to connect deeply with the practice.

2.7. When to Practice

Incorporating yoga and mindfulness into your daily schedule is easier than you think. Morning stretches, evening relaxation poses, or mindful dinners - it's about finding what works best for your family.

The journey of introducing yoga and mindfulness to your family is a transformative one. As each member of your family embarks on it, they learn important life skills such as patience, focus, resilience, and empathy. Remember, yoga is not a race, and neither is mindfulness. They're lifelong skills that grow and mature in due time. In this journey, you'll create countless family moments that, when looked back upon, will bring smiles and warmth to your hearts.

So, here we are, ready to take the first step into a more mindful, present, and active family life. Keep patience, persistence, and thoughtfulness as your companions on this journey. And always remember, it is not about perfect techniques and precision; instead, it's the fun, togetherness, and awareness you cultivate that truly matters.

Chapter 3. Yoga Fundamentals: Basic Postures and Their Benefits

Understanding yoga begins with foundational postures, often referred to as 'asanas' in yogic tradition. Renowned for their numerous health benefits, these basic poses will enhance your flexibility, focus, and overall wellbeing. Moreover, when these postures are properly incorporated into a family setting, they can foster a sense of unity and harmony amongst family members. Let's explore some of these beneficial postures.

3.1. What is an Asana?

'Asana' is a Sanskrit term that translates to 'seat.' In the context of yoga, it refers to the postures or positions used. Asanas teach patience and cultivate concentration, being a stable and comfortable position. There are a multitude of asanas, each with distinct benefits. The fundamental asanas we will explore help lay the foundation for a family yoga practice.

3.2. Tadasana: Mountain Pose

Tadasana, or Mountain Pose, is one of the simplest asanas, and forms the basis for many others.

To practice Tadasana: - Stand tall with feet hip-width apart. - Keep your arms alongside your body, palms facing forward. - Take a deep breath, and raise your hands above your head. - Keep your gaze forward or slightly upward, towards your hands. - Hold this pose for 5-10 breaths, then slowly lower your hands while exhaling.

Tadasana helps improve posture, balance, and self-awareness. It is particularly beneficial for children who are developing their sense of physical coordination.

3.3. Balasana: Child's Pose

Balasana, or Child's Pose, is a calming pose that emulates the fetal position.

To practice Balasana: - Kneel down and sit on your heels. - Lean forward to lay your torso down between your thighs, extending your arms forward. - Rest your forehead on the floor. - Stay in this pose for a few breaths, or longer if comfortable.

This pose is great for relaxation and stress relief. It can be a good way to wind down as a family after a busy day.

3.4. Vrikshasana: Tree Pose

Vrikshasana, or Tree Pose, is an asana that improves balance while strengthening the core and legs.

To practice Vrikshasana: - Start in Tadasana. - Bend your right knee and place your right foot on the inside of your left thigh. - Maintain balance, and once steady, hold your hands together in front of your chest in a prayer position. - For an extra challenge, raise your arms overhead, keeping your gaze forward. - Repeat on the other side.

This pose can be made into a fun balancing challenge for kids.

3.5. Savasana: Corpse Pose

Savasana, or Corpse Pose, provides deep relaxation and is often used to conclude a yoga session.

To practice Savasana: - Lie on your back, with your legs extended and arms alongside your body, palms facing upward. - Close your eyes and breathe deeply and slowly. - Stay in this pose for 5-10 minutes, or until fully relaxed.

This pose can help promote a sense of peace and reduce anxiety, emphasizing the mindfulness aspect of yoga.

These are just a few asanas to get you started on your family yoga journey. Remember, the goal isn't perfection. It's about cultivating mindfulness, patience, and togetherness. Practiced consistently, these poses will contribute to an improved physical health and deeper familial bonds. As you continue, you can explore other asanas and incorporate them into your practice. Moreover, this journey isn't confined to the yoga mat - it extends into everyday life, reminding us of the importance of balance, patience, and understanding. Don't rush the process, enjoy every moment. Namaste!

Chapter 4. Peaceful Parents: Yoga Techniques to Help Navigate Parental Stress

Parenting is a formidable task, and while it brings its own joys and rewards, it also often comes with stress and anxiety. This chapter will take you through a range of yoga techniques that can help you navigate these tense moments with greater tranquility and balance.

4.1. The Landscape of Parental Stress

Before we delve into the yoga techniques, it's essential to first understand the landscape of parental stress. Whether it's the constant worry for your child, the pressure of balancing work and family life, or the strain on relationships, there are many sources of stress that parents often grapple with.

The life of a parent is filled with an assortment of different challenges that change as children grow and develop. From sleepless nights with newborns to managing the unpredictable moods of teenagers, each stage brings unique stresses.

Even as these challenges evolve, remember that you're not alone. Every parent, at some point, will endure the rigors of parenthood. It is these shared trials and tribulations that create the universal understanding among parents.

However, it's your response to this stress that truly shapes your parenting experience. Yoga and its associated mindfulness techniques equip you to handle this stress with grace and equanimity.

4.2. Yoga and Mindfulness: An Introduction

Yoga, a practice rooted in ancient Indian wisdom, is about more than just physical exercise. It is a comprehensive system that unites the mind, body, and spirit, promoting overall health and well-being.

Using a combination of postures (asana), controlled breathing (pranayama), and meditation, yoga fosters deep relaxation, reducing stress and anxiety effectively.

Mindfulness, an integral part of the yoga practice, amplifies these benefits. It is the act of being fully present in the moment, without judgment and without distraction. This state of heightened awareness enables you to observe your emotions and reactions, offering a clearer perspective on situations, thus reducing overreactions or unnecessary stress.

4.3. Yoga Techniques to Alleviate Parental Stress

Let's now dive into the specific yoga techniques which can offer you respite from parental stress, and lead you to embody the essence of a peaceful parent.

4.3.1. Asana Practice: Poses for Peace of Mind

Yoga poses, or asanas, are more than just physical exercises. They are designed to balance the mind and body, opening up energy channels and releasing tension.

1. *Child's Pose (Balasana)*: A comforting pose that emulates the fetal position, Child's Pose allows you to turn within and find calm amidst chaos.

2. *Forward Bend (Uttanasana)*: This pose helps drain away stress, as it improves blood circulation in the brain.

3. *Cow Face Pose (Gomukhasana)*: This seated pose, while challenging, offers deep relaxation as it opens the chest, allowing easier, fuller breaths.

4. *Corpse Pose (Savasana)*: Often concluding a yoga practice, this pose induces deep rest and recuperation.

Remember, the aim is not to perfect these poses but to enjoy the experience they offer. It's more about the journey, rather than the destination.

4.3.2. Pranayama: Breathing Techniques for Stress Relief

Breathing exercises, otherwise known as pranayama, can work as instant stress relievers. Here are a few techniques:

1. *Deep Breathing (Deergha Swasam)*: Deep breathing, done while seated comfortably, involves full, conscious inhalation and exhalation.

2. *Victorious Breath (Ujjayi Pranayama)*: This involves slow inhalation and exhalation, with a slight constriction in the throat, creating a soothing sound like the ocean waves.

3. *Cooling Breath (Sheetali Pranayama)*: This involves inhaling through a rolled tongue and exhaling through the nose. It has a cooling effect on the body.

Remember, when practicing pranayama, ensure you're comfortable and free from distractions.

4.3.3. Meditation and Mindfulness for Parents

Stress often arises when we are caught up in the whirlwind of thoughts about the past or future. Mindfulness brings us back to the present moment, reducing anxiety and stress.

Mindfulness can be cultivated through meditation. Carving out a few minutes every day for meditation can create a significant impact on stress levels. You can begin by simply observing your breath, acknowledging thoughts as they arise, and then gently bringing the focus back to your breath.

4.4. Conclusion: Blending Yoga into Your Daily Routine

Thoughtfully blend your newfound techniques into your daily routine. Perhaps, start your day with a few yoga poses, perform some breathing exercises during lunchtime, and wind down with a small meditation session in the evening.

Refine your practice as you progress, listening to what your body and mind need. Remember, it's not about hard and fast rules, but about cultivating an enjoyable and sustainable practice that helps manage stress and bring about peace and calm.

By practicing these yoga techniques regularly, you will become better equipped to navigate the choppy waters of parental stress, embodying the essence of being a peaceful parent. So unfurl your yoga mat, and set out on this journey to peaceful parenting!

Chapter 5. Weaving Yoga Into Daily Routines: Making Every Moment Count

Remember the frenzy commotion that spins around your household during mornings? Pairing socks, making breakfast, packing lunches, and rushing to the school bus - it usually starts out as a whirlwind. Now, imagine a scenario where you could easily infuse a sense of grounding, balance, and mindfulness even amidst this chaotic whirl. Welcome to our chapter on blending yoga seamlessly into your daily family routines.

5.1. Getting Familiar with Your Yoga Mat

First things first: let's consider the platform upon which we will build our yoga experience - the yoga mat. Your relationship with your mat is crucial, and it will become your sanctuary. Encourage your child to choose their own mat (or create a sacred space) based on color, comfort, or design - something that holds personal appeal for them. This will be their own, personal 'safe space' where they can express, release, and rejuvenate.

It's crucial to make your yoga session amiable. Place your mats side by side, mirroring each other, or create an exciting formation that suits your family's dynamic. The aim is to foster an environment of inclusivity and connection.

5.2. Rise and Shine with Yoga

Rather than hurrying into the flurry of the morning activity, let's start the day by grounding ourselves. A simplified Sun Salutation routine is an exceptional way to affirm the energy of the day, and it's an excellent exercise to induce wakefulness and vitality without straining the body.

1. Start by standing at the edge of your mat, feet apart.

2. Reach your arms upward while taking a deep breath.

3. As you exhale, slowly lean forward from your hips, hands reaching toward the mat.

4. Bring your right foot back into a lunge, while inhaling.

5. Exhale and bring your left foot back, aligning it with your right in a plank pose.

6. Inhale and lower your body to the mat.

7. Exhale and practice Cobra pose – lie flat on your stomach, hands next to your shoulders, lifting the upper body up.

8. Get back on all fours, inhale, and lift your hips towards the ceiling, forming an inverted 'V' or Downward-Facing Dog pose.

9. As you exhale, bring your right foot forward into a lunge.

10. Bring your left foot forward while inhaling, so that you are back in a forward fold.

11. Exhale while slowly rolling up to stand, finishing where you began.

Encourage your young ones to follow your pacing, synchronizing breaths and movements, thus creating a familial rhythm.

5.3. Midday Mini-Moves

Deskwork, studies, and prolonged seated hours can land your body into a stiff mode. To counteract this, use these midday yoga 'mini-moves' to break the stiffness and refresh your energy. They are short, brisk and can fit into any schedule.

1. Try Seated Twists – while sitting, place your right hand on your left knee, twist your upper body to the left, and look over your left shoulder. Repeat on the opposite side.

2. Shoulder Rolls – Roll your shoulders up towards your ears, back, down, and return to the front.

3. Side Stretches – Extend your arms over your head. Holding your right wrist with your left hand, bend to the left. Repeat on the other side.

Remember, these mini-moves are great not only for parents but kids as well. They give a quick break from their study hours, re-energizing them completely.

5.4. The Power of Breath

Teaching children about the power of their breath can bring notable changes to their emotional health. A simple technique like 'Belly Breathing' can help your child manage their emotions and reactions.

1. Begin by sitting or lying down in a comfortable spot.

2. Place one hand on the stomach and the other on the chest.

3. Breathe in slowly through the nose, feel the stomach lift the hand up.

4. Breathe out slowly through the mouth, feel the stomach fall down.

5. Encourage children to imagine the tummy as a balloon which inflates when breathed in and deflates when breathed out.

5.5. Transitioning to Bedtime with Gentle Stretches

Close the day with gentle yoga stretches that pave the way for a good night's sleep. Incorporating peaceful poses like the Child's Pose, Legs-Up-The-Wall Pose, and Happy Baby Pose, can help children wind down and transition to bedtime.

In conclusion, gradually building a practice of intertwining yoga within daily activities takes time and efforts but it has immense benefits. Not only does it help maintain physical health, but it also paves the path for mental well-being. Remember, the aim is not to perform complex poses, but to cultivate mindfulness, resilience, and a sense of inner balance within the family.

Take a deep breath, stretch out the stress, and find your family's unique rhythm.

Chapter 6. Mindful Eating: The Yogic Approach to Family Nutrition

Challenging as it may be to introduce the concept of mindfulness, especially when it comes to food - our deeply conditioned habits, the pace of daily life, and individual preferences all come into play. However, with a gradual and gentle approach, it's possible to bring a profound change in the way you and your family relate to food and nutrition. This section will guide you through the essentials of mindful eating from a yogic perspective and how to establish the same in your family.

6.1. Understanding Mindfulness and Nutrition

Mindfulness is the conscious awareness of one's present moment. Rather than focus on what has happened in the past or may happen in the future, mindful beings live in the 'now', relishing each moment as it unfurls. When applied to eating, mindfulness encourages us to be fully present while consuming our meals, savoring each bite, and appreciating the food that fuels our bodies.

Yogic philosophy aligns beautifully with this concept. One of the central principles of yoga is 'Ahimsa', often translated as non-violence. When it comes to eating, this concept outlines the principles of consuming nourishing food that promotes overall well-being, without causing harm to ourselves or the environment. It too emphasizes the importance of mindful presence while eating, fostering a connection between the body, the mind, and the food.

Moreover, both yoga and the concept of mindful eating shed light on the aspect of Satvic food - food that is pure, clean, and harmonious. Although predominantly vegetarian in accordance with Ahimsa, Satvic food can accommodate individual dietary needs while emphasizing on fruits, vegetables, legumes, nuts, and whole grains produced ethically. It's not just about what we eat, but how we acquire it, prepare it, and consume it.

Let's delve deeper into the intricacies of these topics and their practical application in the subsequent parts of this chapter.

6.2. The Practice of Mindful Eating

Mindful eating is about more than simply slowing down or eating 'healthier.' It is about experiencing food more intensively—especially the pleasure of it. Here are some strategies on how we can encourage ourselves and our children to practice mindful eating:

1. Mindfulness Bites: Before starting your meal, take a moment to feel grateful for your food. Encourage your children to do the same. Now start with small bites, fully aware of each aspect of eating - the color of the food, its aroma, texture, and of course, taste. Savor each bite before reaching for the next one.

2. Eating in Silence: This may seem like a herculean task, especially with kids around, but try to inculcate periods of silence during the mealtime. Even a couple of minutes wherein everyone focuses on their food rather than talking can be tremendously helpful.

3. Ditch Distractions: Make your dining space a 'No-Gadget Zone.' Encourage everyone to leave their phones, tablets, or even books away from the dining table, to fully focus on the meal and the family.

4. Quality over Quantity: Teach your children about the importance of quality over quantity. It's not about filling our plates and stomachs to their maximum capacity but about savoring and

relishing what's on them - a vital lesson in nutrition and satisfaction.

6.3. The Concept of Satvic Food

The term 'Satvic' originates from the Sanskrit word 'Sattva,' meaning pure, virtuous, and peaceful. Satvic diet aims to nurture our bodies and maintain the harmony of our minds. This simple, nutrient-rich diet, predominantly vegetarian, comprises fresh fruits and vegetables, whole grains, dairy products, herbs, nuts, seeds, legumes, and honey.

Yet, the beauty of the Satvic diet is its adaptability. It is not a hard rule but an invitation to make compassionate choices. Therefore, if your family's dietary needs and preferences extend beyond a strictly vegetarian diet, remember the essence of Ahimsa - compassion towards all living beings. Ethically sourced, organic animal products, handled with care and respect for life, can also find a place in the Satvic philosophy.

While considering a predominantly Satvic diet, focus on a few main factors:

1. The Source: Fruits, vegetables, nuts, and grains should be responsibly grown, organic, and GMO-free. Animal-based products, if consumed, should be from ethically treated animals.

2. The Preparation: Cooking should be done with a positive mind and loving hands. This not only makes the food healthier but also infuses positivity.

3. The Consumption: Food should be eaten fresh and in moderate proportions. Overeating, even the most nutritious food, can lead to imbalances in the body.

6.4. Teaching Kids About Nutrition

Nutrition can be a complex subject, especially for children. However, with a compassionate approach, it's possible to blend mindfulness and nutrition, making it a practical and engaging topic for children.

Start with letting them understand the concept of mindful eating first. Once they are habituated, introduce them to the topic of healthy nutrition. Discuss the vitamins, minerals, and other nutrients in their food, their importance, and how these are going to help them grow stronger and healthier. Introduce them to the concept of a balanced meal, representative of the different food groups.

Include children in meal planning and preparation. Let them touch the vegetables, wash the grains, and mix the salad. This hands-on approach can pique their interest and encourage healthier choices.

Finally, let children be children! Allow them a treat now and then to ensure they don't feel overly restricted. Remember, it's balance, not perfection, we're aiming for.

Incorporating yoga and mindful eating in family life isn't always straightforward, yet the rewards are immense. It's not about an overnight transformation but a gradual acceptance of this lifestyle. Involve the entire family in this process, making it a joyful journey for everyone. Remember, yoga is more than the poses; it's a way of life. And what better way to express this than through the way we nourish our bodies and minds - with love, compassion, and mindfulness. Stay patient, stay consistent, and let the magic unfold.

Chapter 7. Mindfulness for Kids: Fun and Easy Techniques for Young Minds

Living mindfully means being present, focusing on the here and now, without judging anything or anyone. It sounds simple, but it's a skill that takes practice both for adults and children, especially in today's fast-paced world. Mindfulness for kids takes these principles and makes them accessible and fun. Teaching your child mindfulness enables them to navigate their feelings better, improve focus, and foster a sense of calm. Let's get started on introducing mindfulness to your little one!

7.1. Understanding Mindfulness for Kids

Before we start practicing mindfulness, it's essential to understand what it means and how kids can benefit. Mindfulness involves paying attention to the current moment, understanding one's feelings and emotions, and accepting oneself without judgment. For kids, this means being fully present during an activity or while interacting with others.

Mindfulness provides various benefits to kids. It helps reduce stress and anxiety, increase self-regulation, and improve concentration and focus. Additionally, mindfulness can assist in developing empathy and understanding towards others, enhancing overall emotional intelligence.

7.2. Why Mindfulness Matters

Earlier, mindfulness works were limited to adults, targeting stress reduction primarily. However, research has pointed out the benefits of mindfulness for kids in recent years. Studies show that it can help improve their performance in school, manage stress and anxiety, and build strong relationships. Moreover, it seeds the qualities of resilience and emotional well-being, helping them navigate through life challenges effectively.

7.3. Introducing Mindfulness to Kids

Start introducing mindfulness by simplifying it to their level. Tell them it's like having a superhero power that helps you see, feel, and understand things, even better. Like how Spiderman uses his 'Spidey Sense', being mindful allows them to use their senses to understand their surroundings and emotions.

7.4. Basic Mindful Techniques For Kids

Here are some simple techniques you can incorporate in your child's routine:

1. Mindful Breathing: Teach your child to focus on their breath. Ask them to take slow, deep breaths, inhaling through their nose and exhaling through their mouth, paying attention to the rise and fall of their chest.

2. Body Scan: This involves paying attention to each part of the body from head to toe. It helps kids understand the connection between their bodies and minds, recognizing tension, and learning to relax.

3. Mindful Eating: Take mealtime as an opportunity to practice

mindfulness. Encourage your child to eat slowly, savoring each bite, noticing the taste, texture, and aroma of the food.

4. Sensory Walk: Arrange a mindful nature walk. Point out the colors, the smells, the sounds, and ask them to describe them. It helps them to stay connected with the environment around them.

7.5. The Mindfulness Jar Activity

An easy and fun mindful activity is creating a mindfulness jar. Fill a jar with glitter and water. Explain to the child as the glitter settles, it's like our mind getting calmer when we sit still and focus. When shaken, the glitter swirling around is like the thoughts in our busy minds.

7.6. Creating a Mindful Environment

A mindful environment at home can help kids adopt the practice more easily. Keep electronic devices away during mindfulness practices. Ensure the area is clear of distractions, creating a quiet and peaceful atmosphere.

In conclusion, mindfulness is a nurturing practice that can facilitate your child's emotional and mental growth. Remember, the key to teaching mindfulness to children is to make it a fun, enjoyable, and rewarding journey. Be patient, and remember it's about progress, not perfection. So, join your kids in this journey and start living the mindful life together!

Chapter 8. Yoga in Motion: Creating Your Family's Flow

Yoga is a practice that engages all levels of your being, from physical to mental and emotional. When you begin to blend your family into this practice, it becomes a way of life that can help you create a sense of unity, harmony, and balance. This chapter outlines ways to build your family's flow through the combination of yoga with daily activities.

8.1. The Road to Harmony

You might be wondering: how should we start? Yoga is often misconceived as a rigid form of exercise, but the truth is, it's about fluidity, motion, and flexibility. You need not change your routine drastically, but rather intertwine yoga into your family's usual activities.

Let's start by incorporating little elements of yoga into your daily tasks. Here are some examples:

- While preparing breakfast, connect with your breath. Take deep inhales as you boil the eggs or pour the cereal, and long exhales as you cut the fruits or toast the bread. Notice how this simple act of mindful breathing calms your mind and sets a serene tone for the day.

- As you send the kids off to school, remind them to stay attentive to their surroundings and mindful of their actions. This is an excellent exercise in present moment awareness or "dharana," a crucial aspect of yoga practice.

- When you finally get some free time as the kids are engaging in activities or studying, roll out your yoga mat for a quick 15-minute yoga session. This "me-time" will not only help you rejuvenate but also subtly introduce this routine into your family's lifestyle.

The focus here is not just the moves or the poses but also the consciousness and the nurturing environment you are creating for your family.

8.2. Embracing Yoga Together

Once you've successfully integrated these small steps into your daily routine, it's time to embrace yoga as a family activity. Here are some creative and engaging ways to introduce the children to the practice:

1. Start with simple yogic breathing exercises. This will help them to become more aware of their bodies and to calm and center their minds.

2. Introduce them to simple poses like the Mountain Pose (Tadasana) or the Warrior Pose (Virabhadrasana). Reiterate that it's not about doing it perfectly, but about experiencing the pose and the moment.

3. Encourage fun and laughter during the sessions. For instance, animal-themed postures such as Cow pose (Bitilasana) or Cat pose (Marjaryasana) can be a hit with younger kids.

4. Create a « Family Yoga » day in your week where all family members participate, each at their own pace.

Remember to always respect everyone's boundaries, and make these sessions a safe space where each family member can relax, unwind and connect.

8.3. Transitioning through the Day

As you become more familiar with yoga, you can start to implement it throughout your day; changing the way you move, react, and incorporate your day's activities. Yoga thus becomes a flowing stream, nurturing your family life.

In the morning, greet the day and your family with a bright smile and a Sun Salutation (Surya Namaskar). This routine can help set a positive tone for the day.

During the day, take short breaks to stretch. Encourage your child to do the same, especially after their online classes or homework. This helps to release tension and rejuvenate the body and mind.

The evening can be your time to unwind and connect. Family yoga sessions, followed by a simple meditation, can be a fantastic way to end the day. You can light candles, play soft music, and let the relaxation of the session seep in, preparing you for a restful night's sleep.

8.4. Creating a Yoga-positive Environment

Amplify the yoga experience by creating a soothing ambiance around you. Bring in green plants, subtle fragrances via essential oils, calming color tones on the walls, and cozy yoga mats. Weaving in these elements not only makes the exercise enjoyable but also triggers the senses, offering a more profound and holistic yoga experience.

Creating your family's flow isn't just about yoga itself; it is about mindfulness, unity, empathy, and balance. It's about respecting individual spaces and energies while also coming together to share and grow as one. Learn, adapt, and find the rhythm that defines and enhances your family's unique lifestyle – your family's yoga-in-motion.

Chapter 9. Coping with Challenge: Using Yoga to Navigate Family Disputes

It is a well-known fact that family conflict can upend the tranquility of a home. Disputes, disagreements, or misunderstandings can seed division and stress within the family. Yoga, however, offers a holistic tool for managing such challenges - invoking not only physical exercises but also mindfulness practice, emotional nurturing and a sense of spiritual unity. This chapter will guide you through the various techniques and strategies to adeptly manage familial discord with yoga as your ally.

9.1. Embracing Mindfulness Amidst Discord

Start by anchoring yourself in the present moment. This simple undertaking, veiled oftentimes by the complexity of our thoughts and emotions, can present a myriad of benefits. Breathe deep, sense your environment, feel your body, notice your thoughts, and simply be aware. Building this practice will help you to remain mindful during tense moments, allowing you to respond with calmness and deliberation instead of reacting impulsively.

Techniques like box-breathing, where you inhale for a count of four, hold for a count of four, exhale for a count of four, and hold once again for a count of four, can induce a profound calmness and focused attention. Practice this during moments of peace, so that when disputes arise, it becomes second nature.

9.2. Transforming Disputes Into Yoga Sessions

Consider turning disagreements into a family yoga session. Begin with a set of gentle poses like 'Mountain Pose' (Tadasana) or 'Tree Pose' (Vriksha-asana). Engage every member into the activity. This will divert the intense energy of the disagreement, providing an environment for peaceful resolution or reflection.

Using yoga during such instances shifts the focus from conflict to cooperation. The flow of the practice calls everyone to work in unison, stimulating empathy and increasing the understanding of each other's strengths and limitations.

9.3. Engages Kids, Encourages Dialogue

Yoga can also provide a communicative platform for younger members of the family. Incorporating playful, animal-themed poses such as 'Downward Dog' (Adho Mukha Svanasana), 'Cobra' (Bhujangasana) or 'Cat-Cow' (Marjaryasana-Bitilasana) can not only spark their interest, but also serve as an opportunity for them to express their feelings.

Maintain an open dialogue throughout the session, asking everyone to share what they feel in each pose. This shared vulnerability can nurture a sense of trust and empathy, promoting a healthier way to address disputes.

9.4. Body Posture and Emotional States

Our body posture impacts our emotional state, and vice-versa. In situations of conflict, our bodies typically close up, representing a defensive state. Through yoga, one can consciously adjust these postures, thereby influencing emotional responses.

Practicing expansive poses like 'Warrior' (Virabhadrasana) and 'Cobra' (Bhujangasana) can give a sense of security and confidence, while positions like 'Child's pose' (Balasana) provide comfort and ease. Bring these poses into your family's routine, giving everyone the tools to self-regulate their emotions consciously.

9.5. Amidst Tensions, Breathing Counts

When engaged in conflicts, we often hold our breath or resort to shallow breathing without noticing. This kind of breathing potentiates the fight-or-flight response, exacerbating the conflict. Use pranayama, the practice of breath control, to counteract this response.

Practicing 'Equal Breathing' (Sama Vritti) or 'Belly Breathing' (Diaphragmatic breathing) can help resist emotional overwhelm during moments of heated family dispute. They impart a measure of control over your physiological responses, helping to calm your mind and dampen reactive impulses.

9.6. The Practice of Compassion Through Shared Yoga

Implement the practice of partner or group yoga poses like 'Double Tree' (Dwi Vriksha-asana) or 'Group Boat' (Navasana) that require synchronisation and cooperation. This nurtures a sense of shared ordeal and encourages empathetic communication.

This can transform a negative situation into a constructive one, breaking the cycle of argument or confrontation, and allowing an environment of compassion and mutual understanding to flourish.

9.7. Investing in Daily Practice

The benefits accrued from the regular practice of yoga aren't restricted to times of family disputes. They also contribute positively to personal growth and family harmony on a daily basis. A family that practices yoga together tends to communicate more effectively, demonstrating increased understanding and reduced interpersonal friction.

The techniques discussed in this chapter are not intended as standalone solutions for deep-seated family issues, which may also require professional help. They should be seen as part of a palette of methods for fostering a more harmonious, understanding, and compassionate family environment, where disputes become opportunities for growth rather than sources of division.

Chapter 10. Bedtime Bliss: Yoga Techniques for Better Sleep

In many households, bedtime can be a battleground, marked by negotiations, pleas, and rebukes. Or maybe it's just a hectic rush, piled between dinner chaos, last-minute homework, and that never-ending pile of laundry. However, it doesn't have to be this way. Yoga, with its focus on mindfulness and relaxation, can become a vessel to more tranquil evenings and better sleep for all.

10.1. Integrating Yoga into Bedtime Routine

Creating a routine that incorporates mindfulness and movement is an excellent first step toward peaceful slumbers. Allow room for a few minutes of yoga before bedtime. To facilitate tranquility, dim the lights and create a calm ambiance. You could also play soft, soothing music in the background to help set the tone.

Start by having a discussion with your children about why sleep is essential-instilling the idea that sleep is not a punishment, but rather a time for their bodies to rest, recharge, and grow. Tie this in with the purpose of yoga — explaining how yoga exercises can help them relax and enjoy a more restful sleep.

10.2. Yoga Poses for Better Sleep

The following yoga postures can be incorporated into your bedtime routine with ease. Ensure they are performed on a comfortable surface like a yoga mat or carpet. Remember, the main goal is to promote relaxation rather than athleticism.

- *Child's Pose (Balasana)*: Kneel on the floor, sit on your heels, and lean forward with your arms stretched out in front. Rest your forehead on the floor. Child's pose is a restorative pose that helps to relax the body and mind.

- *Legs-Up-the-Wall Pose (Viparita Karani)*: Lie on your back close to a wall. Extend your legs straight up against the wall. This pose can reduce stress levels and help to calm the mind.

- *Supine Twists*: Lie on your back, hug your knees into your chest, then drop both knees over to one side. Look over the opposite shoulder to complete the spinal twist. Switch sides. This pose promotes relaxation and assists in calming the nervous system.

- *Corpse Pose (Savasana)*: Lie flat on your back with your arms and legs comfortably extended. Close your eyes and take deep, slow breaths. Savasana is a restorative asana that helps to center the mind and relax the body, preparing it for sleep.

10.3. Mindful Breathing for Soothing Sleep

Breathing exercises, or Pranayama, are an integral aspect of yoga that can be particularly beneficial when preparing for sleep. These exercises can teach children (and adults, too!) how to control their breath, manage stress, and soothe themselves to sleep.

1. *Belly Breathing*: Have your child lie on their back. Place a stuffed animal on their belly. As they breathe in, the stuffed animal will rise, and as they exhale, it will lower. This simple technique can help calm the mind and body.

2. *Bumblebee Breath (Bhramari Pranayama)*: In this breathing exercise, everyone hums like a bee while exhaling. The vibrations can have a calming effect, aiding in better sleep.

3. *4-7-8 Breathing*: Inhale for a count of four, hold your breath for a count of seven, and exhale for a count of eight. The aim of this exercise is to slow down the breath, allowing for deep relaxation.

10.4. Progressive Muscle Relaxation for Better Sleep

Progressive Muscle Relaxation (PMR) is a technique that involves tensing and relaxing muscle groups throughout the body, helping to promote relaxation and sleep. Here is a step-by-step guide on how to practice PMR with children:

1. Sit or lie down comfortably.

2. Start with the toes. Instruct your kids to squeeze their toes tight and then release.

3. Move up to the legs. Tighten the leg muscles, hold, and then relax.

4. Continue through the body — the belly, hands, arms, shoulders, and face.

The tightening and releasing sensation helps create awareness of the body's state of tension or relaxation, ultimately promoting enhanced sleep quality.

10.5. Conclusion: The Power of Continuity

Consistency is the secret to success when integrating yoga techniques into your bedtime routine. Regularity cultivates familiarity, providing psychological comfort and familiarity, which can promote better sleep. Moreover, it's essential to adjust and adapt these suggestions to fit your family's needs and schedules. Personalizing your routine will make it more enjoyable, leading to increased adherence and, ultimately, a longer, sounder sleep.

Savor these quiet, bonding moments with your children. Through yoga, you teach them valuable skills for relaxation and mindfulness — benefits that extend well beyond a good night's sleep. This is a beautiful way to conclude your day, inviting tranquility into your family life, one mindful moment and deep breath at a time.

Chapter 11. Celebrating Progress: Creating a Family Yoga Journal and Articulating Milestones

Documenting the journey of implementing yoga into your family's routine can be a personal and appealing way to track progress, celebrate milestones, and fuel motivations. In this chapter, we will guide you through the entire process of creating a captivating Family Yoga Journal, as well as articulating and commemorating milestones with your loved ones.

11.1. Initiating Your Family Yoga Journal

Start by selecting a journal that fits your family's style and needs. It could be a spiral-bound notebook, an artistically decorated diary, or even an online blog. Whatever the medium, it must resonate with your family and invite you to dedicate time in sharing your thoughts, emotions, and experiences.

Your Family Yoga Journal is an interactive playground. Here, you can note down reflections on your yoga sessions, list out your favorite poses, draw doodles depicting memorable moments, and paste photographs of your family practicing yoga.

11.2. Transforming Observations into Entries

It can be helpful to break down your observations into three categories: Body, Mind, and Spirit. After each yoga session, take a moment to reflect on these three areas.

1. Body: How do your physical selves feel after the session? Document any noticeable changes in flexibility, strength, or balance.

2. Mind: How did the session impact your mental state? Were you able to shake off stress, to find clarity in your thoughts, or to become more focused?

3. Spirit: Did the session touch your soul in any way? Did it induce a sense of peace, love, joy, or other uplifting emotions?

Incorporate your observations into your journal entries to create a holistic view of your family's yoga journey.

11.3. Celebrating Progress and Articulating Milestones

Tracking progress is an essential aspect of motivation when practicing yoga as a family. It not only provides a tangible measure of your achievements but also reminds you that every small step you take contributes to your yoga journey.

Record your initial capabilities when you first start practicing yoga: how long each of you could maintain a pose, the forms you could perform successfully, or your breathing patterns. As time goes by, you will notice improvements in these areas, and your journal will act as a consistent milestone tracker - a token of your collective hard work and persistence.

11.4. Incorporating Artistic Expression

Art can be a wonderful means to express one's feelings, thoughts, and experiences. Encourage every member of the family to draw, paint or even sculpt to depict their yoga journey. Do not limit this to literal representations; abstract art can beautifully capture emotions and sensations. You can then include this artwork in your journal, adding a touch of creativity and personalization to your record.

11.5. Encouraging Heartfelt Reflections

A Family Yoga Journal should be more than just a log of yoga practices; it can also host a treasury of heartfelt reflections. Encourage each family member to write about their experiences. They can compose poems, stories, or essays that reflect on their personal yoga journey.

11.6. Bringing it Together: Co-creating the Journal

Remember, this is a Family Yoga Journal, a merging of individual journeys into a unified narrative. Ensure each member contributes, creates, and co-authors the contents. The journal will then become a symbol of your shared journey, your shared growth, and your shared bond. It will stand testament to your collective pursuit of mindfulness, movement, and harmony.

Each page turned becomes a milestone achieved, and every session added anew will become a memento to look back on - a reflection of a happy, healthy, and harmonious family honoring the spirit of yoga together.

As you regularly engage with your Family Yoga Journal, you'll find the practice promoting appreciation for progress, gratitude for shared experiences, and a joyous anticipation of the milestones still to be reached.